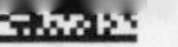

BODY BUILDING WORKOUT GUIDE FOR AGES 40 AND ABOVE

Unleashing Vitality, Defying Limits, and Crafting Your Ageless Legacy in the World of Bodybuilding Mastery

Raymond M. Arnold

TABLE OF CONTENT

I. Introduction

Welcome to the Bodybuilding Workout Plan for Men Above 40! This comprehensive guide has been meticulously crafted to address the unique fitness needs and considerations of individuals in the age group of 40 and above. As we embark on this journey, it is crucial to recognize the distinct requirements that come with age and to design a workout plan that fosters strength, resilience, and overall well-being.

A. Purpose of the Workout Plan

The primary goal of this workout plan is to empower men above 40 with a structured and effective approach to bodybuilding. We understand that this stage in life may bring about changes in metabolism, recovery rates, and potential limitations, and our plan is tailored to accommodate these factors. Whether you're a seasoned fitness enthusiast or just beginning your journey, this plan is designed to enhance muscular strength, promote cardiovascular health, and optimize overall functional fitness.

B. Considerations for Men Above 40

Age brings both wisdom and unique challenges, and our workout plan takes into account the importance of joint health, injury prevention, and gradual progress. We emphasize the significance of consulting with a healthcare professional before commencing this program, ensuring that your fitness journey aligns with your individual health status and goals.

C. Importance of Consulting a Healthcare Professional

Before embarking on any new fitness regimen, especially for individuals above 40, consulting with a healthcare professional is paramount. This ensures that the workout plan is adapted to your specific health conditions and helps identify any potential risks. Your safety and well-being are our top priorities, and we encourage you to take this crucial step before diving into the workouts outlined in this guide.

Prepare to embark on a transformative fitness journey that goes beyond building muscle—it's about fostering a sustainable and healthy lifestyle. Let's elevate your fitness, enhance your vitality, and redefine what it means to thrive in the prime of life.

II. Warm-up and Mobility

A. Importance of Warm-up

The Tale of John's Awakening

Meet John, a 42-year-old executive who, like many in his age group, led a busy and sedentary lifestyle. One day, determined to reclaim his health, John decided to embark on a fitness journey. Excited but cautious, he joined a gym and met with a personal trainer, Sarah.

Sarah shared a story with John about another client named Mike, who had skipped warm-ups due to time constraints. Mike, in his eagerness to lift heavy weights, suffered an injury that set back his progress and left him frustrated. Learning from Mike's experience, John understood the importance of a proper warm-up.

B. Dynamic Stretching

The Yoga Master's Secret

Incorporating dynamic stretching into the warm-up routine, John learned about a yoga master,

Richard, who celebrated his 50th birthday with remarkable flexibility and strength. Richard attributed his agility to years of consistent dynamic stretching, which not only prepared his muscles for intense workouts but also improved his overall mobility. John, inspired by Richard's story, embraced dynamic stretching as an essential part of his warm-up.

C. Joint Mobility Exercises

The Marathoner's Wisdom

Sarah shared the story of Lisa, a 45-year-old marathon runner who swore by joint mobility exercises. Despite the pounding her joints took during long-distance runs, Lisa remained injury-free due to her diligent focus on joint health. John realized that incorporating joint mobility exercises not only increased flexibility but also acted as a preventative measure against potential injuries—key for someone in their 40s and beyond.

In this chapter, we delve into the stories of individuals like John, Mike, Richard, and Lisa to underscore the significance of warm-up and mobility. Each narrative serves as a reminder that a few extra minutes invested in preparing the body can make a substantial difference in the long-term success of a fitness journey.

So, as you lace up your sneakers and prepare to embark on the exercises outlined in the following chapters, remember the lessons from these stories. A well-executed warm-up and mobility routine isn't just a prelude to your workout; it's a foundation for a resilient, injury-resistant, and enduring fitness experience.

III. Resistance Training

Embark on the transformative journey of Resistance Training, a cornerstone of our bodybuilding workout plan for men above 40. This chapter is your roadmap to sculpting a robust physique, enhancing muscular strength, and embracing the empowering benefits of lifting weights.

A. Overview of Resistance Training

Unleashing Your Inner Strength: Discover the profound impact of resistance training on your body and mind. From building lean muscle mass to fortifying bones, resistance training is the catalyst for transformation. Dive into the science behind resistance exercises and understand how they form the bedrock of your fitness expedition.

B. Choosing Appropriate Weights

Precision in Progression: In the pursuit of strength, selecting the right weights is an art. Learn the nuances of choosing weights that challenge without compromising form. Explore the dynamic interplay between intensity and sustainability, ensuring each rep propels you toward your goals, fostering growth while mitigating the risk of injury.

C. Full Body Workouts vs. Split Routines

Strategic Approaches to Sculpting: Navigate the dichotomy between full-body workouts and split routines. Tailor your training approach to align with your lifestyle and goals. Uncover the benefits of comprehensive full-body engagement or the targeted focus of split routines, all within the context of optimizing results for the seasoned warrior above 40.

D. Workout Phases

Embark on a multi-phased odyssey designed to guide you through progressive levels of strength and muscular development.

1. Phase 1: Foundation Building (4-6 weeks)

Laying the Groundwork: Initiate your journey with compound exercises that form the bedrock of strength. Discover the synergy between reps, sets, and rest intervals, establishing a solid foundation for the challenges ahead.

2. Phase 2: Strength Development (6-8 weeks)

The Power Within: Elevate your strength game through progressive overload and innovative intensity techniques. Delve into strategies for optimal recovery, ensuring your body evolves into a resilient powerhouse.

3. Phase 3: Hypertrophy and Definition (8-10 weeks)

Chisel Your Masterpiece: Fine-tune your physique with targeted approaches to hypertrophy. Explore rep ranges that stimulate muscle growth and unveil strategies for cutting, revealing the sculpted masterpiece beneath.

Empower yourself through the art and science of resistance training. Your body is a canvas; let each lift and rep be a brushstroke, shaping the masterpiece of strength and vitality that is uniquely yours.

IV. Workout Phases

A. Phase 1: Foundation Building (4-6 weeks)

1. Compound Exercises

In the initial phase of your workout plan, emphasis will be placed on compound exercises. These movements engage multiple muscle groups simultaneously, laying a solid foundation for overall strength and muscle development. Squats, deadlifts, and bench presses will be your allies in building a robust physique.

2. Reps and Sets

Understanding the right balance between repetitions and sets is crucial. During the foundation-building phase, a moderate rep range (8-12 reps) and multiple sets will stimulate muscle growth without compromising form. This approach ensures gradual adaptation and minimizes the risk of overtraining.

3. Rest Periods

Allowing adequate rest between sets is often underestimated. While intensity is essential, proper rest intervals (around 60-90 seconds) strike a balance between challenging your muscles and facilitating recovery. This approach optimizes the efficiency of your workouts, ensuring consistent progress.

B. Phase 2: Strength Development (6-8 weeks)

1. Progressive Overload

The second phase introduces the concept of progressive overload. To stimulate continuous muscle growth, gradually increase the resistance you lift. This could involve adding weight, increasing repetitions, or adjusting the intensity of your exercises. Progressive overload challenges your muscles, fostering strength gains over time.

2. Introducing Intensity Techniques

To break through plateaus and keep your workouts dynamic, introduce intensity techniques. Techniques such as drop sets, supersets, and pyramids add variety to your routine, enhancing muscle stimulation and promoting further strength development.

3. Recovery Strategies

Recognizing the importance of recovery is paramount. In this phase, strategic rest days, proper sleep, and nutritional support become critical. These recovery strategies ensure that your body can adapt to the increased demands, minimizing the risk of overtraining and enhancing overall workout effectiveness.

C. Phase 3: Hypertrophy and Definition (8-10 weeks)

1. Targeting Specific Muscle Groups

As you progress, focus on targeting specific muscle groups for hypertrophy. Tailoring your workouts to emphasize muscle development in key areas will contribute to a well-defined and proportionate physique.

2. Hypertrophy Rep Ranges

Adjusting rep ranges to favor hypertrophy (around 6-10 reps) maximizes muscle size and definition. This phase emphasizes controlled, deliberate movements to effectively target the muscle fibers responsible for growth.

3. Cutting Strategies for Definition

The final weeks of the plan incorporate cutting strategies to reveal your hard-earned muscle definition. Adjusting your nutrition, incorporating cardio, and refining your workout routine will help shed excess body fat while preserving muscle mass.

In this phase-based approach, each stage serves a specific purpose in your bodybuilding journey. Whether you're building a foundation, enhancing strength, or refining definition, these practical guidelines ensure a systematic and effective progression toward your fitness goals.

V. Cardiovascular Exercise

A. Importance of Cardiovascular Health

Cardiovascular exercise, often referred to as cardio, plays a pivotal role in the overall fitness journey for men above 40. Beyond the aesthetic benefits, it significantly contributes to heart health, stamina, and overall well-being.

1. *Heart Health and Longevity*

Cardiovascular exercises, such as running, cycling, and swimming, are renowned for enhancing heart health. Engaging in regular cardio workouts strengthens the heart muscle, improves blood circulation, and lowers the risk of cardiovascular diseases. Consider it an investment in your longevity and a proactive measure against age-related health issues.

2. *Weight Management and Metabolism Boost*

For many men above 40, maintaining a healthy weight becomes a priority. Cardio exercises are effective in burning calories and aiding weight management. Moreover, cardio boosts metabolism, helping your body efficiently utilize energy and combat the natural slowdown that can come with age.

B. Suitable Cardio Activities

Choosing the right cardio activities is crucial to ensure engagement and sustainability in your fitness routine.

1. *Low-Impact Options*

Consider low-impact exercises like brisk walking, elliptical training, or swimming. These activities are gentler on the joints, reducing the risk of injuries, a factor that becomes increasingly important as we age.

2. *Interval Training for Efficiency*

Incorporating interval training, alternating between high-intensity bursts and recovery periods, can be a time-efficient yet highly effective way to boost cardiovascular fitness. This approach accommodates busy schedules while maximizing the benefits of cardio workouts.

C. Frequency and Duration

1. Consistency Over Intensity

Consistency trumps intensity, especially for individuals above 40. Aim for at least 150 minutes of moderate-intensity aerobic activity or 75 minutes of vigorous-intensity aerobic activity per week, spread across most days. Consistent, moderate efforts are sustainable and yield lasting benefits.

2. Listening to Your Body

Listen to your body signals. If you're just starting or returning to cardio after a hiatus, gradually increase the duration and intensity. Pay attention to how your body responds and be mindful of any discomfort or signs of overtraining.

In this chapter, we delve into the practical aspects of cardiovascular exercise, emphasizing its crucial role in maintaining health, managing weight, and enhancing overall fitness for men above 40. The key lies not only in the type of cardio chosen but also in the consistency and mindfulness applied to each session.

VI. Flexibility and Mobility

A. Stretching for Flexibility

1. Dynamic Stretching Essentials

Flexibility isn't just for yogis; it's a crucial component for anyone looking to improve their overall fitness, especially for men above 40. Dynamic stretching, involving controlled, full-range-of-motion movements, plays a pivotal role in enhancing flexibility. Picture this: imagine your muscles as rubber bands. Without proper stretching, they can become tight and less pliable. Dynamic stretching helps to extend those rubber bands, promoting flexibility and preparing your body for the demands of the workout.

2. The Power of Static Stretching

Static stretching, while often debated, finds its place in our plan when performed at the right time. Consider it as a tool to improve your range of motion and flexibility further. Hold those stretches for 15-30 seconds, focusing on key muscle groups. As you consistently incorporate static stretching into your routine, you'll notice increased flexibility and improved muscle function over time.

B. Yoga and Pilates

1. Yoga for Strength and Flexibility

Yoga isn't just about striking poses; it's a powerful tool for building strength, balance, and flexibility. The controlled movements and focused breathing promote a mind-body connection, enhancing overall well-being. Incorporating yoga into your routine can improve your flexibility while providing a mental respite from the daily grind. It's a holistic approach that aligns seamlessly with the goals of our workout plan.

2. Pilates for Core Stability

Pilates is another gem in our flexibility arsenal. Beyond its reputation for sculpting a lean physique, Pilates focuses on core strength and stability. A strong core is the foundation for good posture and efficient movement. As men age, maintaining core strength becomes increasingly vital. Pilates exercises, with their emphasis on controlled movements, help achieve this, contributing to improved flexibility and reduced risk of injuries.

C. Foam Rolling and Self-Myofascial Release

1. The Role of Foam Rolling

Ever felt those knots in your muscles after an intense workout? Enter foam rolling, a form of self-myofascial release. Foam rolling helps release tension in the fascia, the connective tissue surrounding muscles. It's like giving your muscles a massage, promoting blood flow and reducing muscle tightness. Integrating foam rolling into your post-workout routine can enhance flexibility, aid recovery, and keep your muscles in prime condition.

2. The DIY Massage with Self-Myofascial Release Techniques

Imagine having the power to perform a DIY massage to soothe tired muscles. That's the beauty of self-myofascial release techniques, utilizing tools like lacrosse balls or massage sticks to target specific areas of tightness. These techniques enhance flexibility, break down adhesions, and contribute to overall muscle health. By incorporating self-myofascial release into your routine, you're actively participating in your body's recovery process.

In this chapter, we explore the practical aspects of flexibility and mobility. From dynamic stretching to yoga, Pilates, foam rolling, and self-myofascial release, these techniques are not mere add-ons but integral components that elevate your fitness journey. By embracing flexibility and mobility practices, you're not just preparing your body for the workout; you're investing in its longevity and resilience.

VII. Recovery and Rest

A. Sleep and its Impact on Recovery

The Sleep Revolution of Tom

Meet Tom, a 48-year-old IT professional struggling with fatigue and lack of progress in his fitness journey. Tom's breakthrough came when he prioritized sleep. Learning from his experience, we explore the transformative power of quality sleep on muscle recovery, hormone regulation, and cognitive function. Tom's commitment to consistent, restorative sleep became the cornerstone of his rejuvenated fitness routine.

B. Active Recovery Days

The Tale of the Weekend Warrior

Imagine Jake, a 44-year-old weekend warrior, whose passion for intense workouts left him fatigued and prone to injuries. Sarah introduced Jake to the concept of active recovery days. Jake discovered that activities like leisurely cycling or gentle yoga on these days not only sped up recovery but also enhanced his overall performance during more intense workouts. Jake's story demonstrates that strategic rest doesn't mean stagnation; it's an active process fueling long-term gains.

C. Incorporating Rest Weeks

Lisa's Strategic Pause

Lisa, a 46-year-old fitness enthusiast, reached a plateau despite her consistent efforts. Sarah guided Lisa through the importance of planned rest weeks. Lisa's initially reluctant decision to dial back her training paid off, leading to improved strength and endurance. Her story underscores that periodic rest is not a setback but a strategic move that allows the body to recharge, preventing burnout and promoting sustained progress.

In this chapter, we uncover the stories of Tom, Jake, and Lisa to emphasize the critical role of recovery and rest in the fitness journey for men above 40. The narratives offer practical insights into the transformative effects of prioritizing sleep, embracing active recovery, and strategically incorporating rest weeks.

As you read on, remember that recovery is not a sign of weakness; it's a strategic weapon in the arsenal of a seasoned fitness enthusiast. So, let these stories inspire you to embrace the power of rest, allowing your body to recover, adapt, and emerge stronger than ever.

VIII. Nutrition and Hydration

A. Importance of Balanced Nutrition

Fueling Your Body for Performance

Meet Mark, a 48-year-old fitness enthusiast who, after years of inconsistent nutrition, decided to revamp his diet for optimal performance. Mark's journey teaches us the importance of balanced nutrition as the cornerstone of any successful bodybuilding plan.

Mark's initial approach was solely focused on protein intake, thinking it would be the magic bullet for muscle growth. However, he soon discovered that a well-rounded diet was essential for sustained energy levels, recovery, and overall health.

1. **Protein's Role in Muscle Health:** Mark learned that while protein is crucial for muscle repair and growth, a balanced approach is key. His diet now includes lean meats, dairy, eggs, and plant-based protein

sources, ensuring a diverse amino acid profile that supports muscle health.

2. **Carbohydrates for Energy:** Recognizing the importance of carbohydrates, Mark incorporated complex carbs like whole grains, fruits, and vegetables into his meals. Carbs became his primary energy source, fueling intense workouts and aiding in post-exercise recovery.

3. **Healthy Fats for Hormonal Balance:** Through trial and error, Mark discovered the significance of incorporating healthy fats into his diet. Nuts, avocados, and olive oil became staples, contributing to hormonal balance, joint health, and overall well-being.

4. **Micronutrients and Antioxidants:** Mark's journey taught him that vitamins and minerals are essential for various bodily functions. Colorful fruits and vegetables filled his plate, providing a spectrum of micronutrients and

antioxidants that support immune function and reduce inflammation.

As we navigate the landscape of balanced nutrition, Mark's story emphasizes that a holistic approach is key. It's not just about macronutrient ratios but also about embracing a variety of nutrient-dense foods for comprehensive health and vitality.

B. Protein Intake for Muscle Health

The Case of Steve's Protein Journey

Steve, a 44-year-old fitness enthusiast, found himself overwhelmed by conflicting information about protein intake. Through his experiences, we uncover the nuanced approach to protein consumption for optimal muscle health.

1. **Individualized Protein Needs:** Steve learned that the ideal protein intake varies based on factors such as body weight, activity level, and fitness goals. Consulting with a nutritionist helped him determine his personalized protein requirements,

ensuring he met the needs of his body without excess.

2. **Timing and Distribution:** Understanding the importance of protein timing, Steve adopted a strategy of distributing protein intake across his meals. This approach not only enhanced muscle protein synthesis but also provided a steady release of amino acids throughout the day.

3. **Supplementation Considerations:** Steve's journey shed light on the role of protein supplements. While he incorporated protein shakes for convenience, he realized that whole food sources offered additional benefits such as fiber and micronutrients.

4. **Hydration's Impact on Protein Utilization:** Steve discovered the interplay between hydration and protein utilization. Proper fluid intake improved digestion, nutrient absorption, and the overall

efficiency of protein utilization within the body.

Steve's experience underscores that achieving optimal muscle health requires a tailored approach to protein intake—one that aligns with individual needs and complements the broader nutritional strategy.

C. Hydration Guidelines

Emma's Journey to Hydration Mastery

Meet Emma, a 41-year-old fitness enthusiast, whose journey highlights the critical role of hydration in overall health and workout performance.

1. **Water as a Performance Enhancer:** Emma realized that dehydration can significantly impact exercise performance. Through trial and error, she identified her optimal water intake, ensuring she remained adequately hydrated before, during, and after workouts.

2. **Electrolyte Balance:** Emma's story emphasizes the importance of maintaining electrolyte balance, especially during intense workouts. Incorporating electrolyte-rich foods and, when needed, sports drinks, helped her prevent dehydration-related issues like cramping and fatigue.

3. **Timing Hydration with Workouts:** Emma learned that strategic hydration enhances workout efficiency. Pre-hydration, sipping water during exercise, and rehydration post-workout became integral parts of her routine, optimizing performance and recovery.

4. **Individual Variability:** Emma's journey highlighted that hydration needs vary among individuals. Factors such as climate, exercise intensity, and individual sweat rates play a role in determining the optimal amount of fluid intake.

Emma's experience serves as a reminder that hydration is not a one-size-fits-all concept. By paying attention to your body's signals and adjusting your fluid intake accordingly, you can optimize your performance and well-being.

In this exploration of nutrition and hydration, the stories of Mark, Steve, and Emma showcase the personalized nature of dietary choices. It's not just about following generic guidelines but about understanding your body's unique needs and crafting a nutrition plan that fuels your individual journey.

IX. Supplements

A. Overview of Common Supplements

Navigating the Supplement Landscape

As our bodies age, meeting nutritional demands solely through diet can become challenging. This chapter explores the role of supplements in enhancing the effectiveness of your bodybuilding journey. Before delving into specific supplements, it's crucial to understand that these should complement, not replace, a balanced diet.

1. **Multivitamins:** Multivitamins provide a convenient way to fill potential nutrient gaps. Men above 40 commonly benefit from supplements containing vitamins A, C, D, E, and K, along with essential minerals like zinc and selenium. These nutrients play vital roles in immune function, bone health, and overall well-being.

2. **Omega-3 Fatty Acids:** Omega-3 supplements, rich in EPA and DHA, contribute to joint health, cardiovascular

function, and anti-inflammatory responses. Sources include fish oil, algae oil for plant-based options, and flaxseed oil.

3. **Calcium and Vitamin D:** To support bone health, especially important as we age, consider a calcium supplement paired with vitamin D for optimal absorption. This combination contributes to bone density and reduces the risk of fractures.

4. **Protein Supplements:** While whole foods should be the primary protein source, supplements like whey protein can be convenient post-workout options. They provide a quick and easily digestible source of essential amino acids.

5. **Creatine:** Creatine enhances muscle strength, aids in recovery, and supports cognitive function. It's a naturally occurring compound found in small amounts in animal products. Creatine monohydrate is a common and well-researched form.

B. Supplements for Joint Health

The Curious Case of Vitamin C and Joint Resilience

Joint health becomes increasingly important as we age, and Vitamin C plays a pivotal role in collagen synthesis—a crucial component of joint structure.

1. **Vitamin C's Role:** Vitamin C is vital for the formation of collagen, which provides strength and elasticity to tendons, ligaments, and cartilage. A deficiency can lead to joint pain and impaired recovery.

2. **Supplement Preparation:** While whole foods like citrus fruits, strawberries, and bell peppers are excellent sources of Vitamin C, supplements can provide an additional boost. Consider a Vitamin C supplement with bioflavonoids, which enhance its absorption.

3. **Glucosamine and Chondroitin:** These supplements are popular for promoting

joint health. Glucosamine supports the formation of cartilage, while chondroitin helps maintain its elasticity. Combining them provides comprehensive support for joint function.

4. **Preparing Joint Health Supplements:** When supplementing with glucosamine and chondroitin, consistency is key. Consider dividing the recommended dose throughout the day to maintain a steady supply in your system.

C. Consultation with a Nutritionist

Tailoring Supplements to Your Individual Needs

1. **Nutritionist's Expertise:** Consulting with a nutritionist ensures that your supplement regimen aligns with your specific needs and health goals. They can assess your dietary intake, identify potential deficiencies, and recommend personalized supplements.

2. **Blood Tests:** Periodic blood tests can provide valuable insights into your nutrient levels. A nutritionist, alongside your healthcare provider, can interpret these results and make informed recommendations.

3. **Adjusting Dosages:** Individual responses to supplements can vary. A nutritionist can help fine-tune dosages based on your body's unique requirements, ensuring you receive optimal benefits without unnecessary excess.

4. **Integrating Supplements into Your Diet:** Your nutritionist will guide you on seamlessly incorporating supplements into your daily routine. Whether it's taking them with meals or at specific times, their expertise ensures maximal absorption and effectiveness.

In this exploration of supplements, we've uncovered their potential contributions to your bodybuilding journey. Remember, supplements are meant to complement a well-rounded diet, not replace it. By understanding the specific vitamins involved and how to prepare and integrate these supplements, you can optimize their benefits and support your fitness goals effectively.

X. Monitoring Progress

A. Keeping a Workout Journal

The Power of Daily Logs

1. **Setting the Foundation:** Start by documenting your current fitness level, including key metrics like weight, body measurements, and strength benchmarks. This establishes a baseline against which you can track progress.

2. **Workout Details:** Log each workout, noting exercises, sets, reps, and weights used. This allows you to monitor strength gains, identify patterns, and make informed adjustments to your training program.

3. **Energy Levels and Recovery:** Record how you feel before, during, and after workouts. Note energy levels, any signs of fatigue, and the quality of your recovery. This insight helps optimize training frequency and intensity.

4. **Nutrition Tracking:** Include details about your daily nutrition. Document meals, water intake, and supplement usage. This comprehensive view helps identify correlations between dietary habits and performance.

B. Tracking Strength and Endurance

Daily Schedules for Optimal Performance

1. **Strategic Workout Timing:** Align your workouts with peak energy levels. Some individuals prefer morning sessions for a kickstart to the day, while others find their strength peaks in the afternoon or evening. Experiment and find what suits you best.

2. **Balancing Intensity and Recovery:** Schedule high-intensity workouts on days when you can prioritize recovery. Consider your work and life commitments to avoid consecutive days of intense training without adequate rest.

3. **Incorporating Active Recovery Days:** Dedicate specific days to active recovery. This could involve light exercises, mobility work, or activities like yoga. Active recovery enhances circulation, reduces muscle stiffness, and contributes to overall well-being.

C. Adjusting the Plan as Needed

The Art of Flexibility in Planning

1. **Listening to Your Body:** Regularly assess how your body responds to training and adjust accordingly. If you're consistently fatigued or experiencing persistent soreness, it might be time for a brief break or a deload week.

2. **Periodization for Long-Term Success:** Implement periodization in your training plan. This involves varying the intensity and volume over specific periods to prevent plateaus and enhance overall performance.

3. **Goal Reassessment:** Periodically reassess your fitness goals. As you age and progress, priorities may shift. Adjust your training plan to align with your evolving objectives, whether it's strength gains, endurance improvements, or overall health.

4. **Consultation with Fitness Professionals:** If unsure about adjustments, seek guidance from a fitness professional. They can provide an objective perspective, assess your progress, and recommend modifications to keep your workouts effective and engaging.

D. Comprehensive Daily Plan

A Day in the Life of a Bodybuilder Above 40

1. **Morning Routine:**
   - Begin your day with dynamic stretching or a short yoga session.
   - Consume a balanced breakfast with protein, complex carbs, and healthy fats.

- Consider taking essential supplements based on your nutritionist's recommendations.

2. **Work and Life Integration:**
   - Schedule your workout during a time that aligns with your energy peaks.
   - Incorporate short breaks throughout the day for mobility exercises or a brisk walk to maintain energy levels and focus.

3. **Post-Workout Nutrition:**
   - Consume a post-workout meal rich in protein and carbohydrates to support recovery.
   - Stay hydrated, considering additional electrolyte intake if needed, especially during intense workouts.

4. **Evening Routine:**
   - Reflect on your daily journal entries, assessing how your body responded to training, nutrition, and overall stress levels.
   - Prepare a nutritious dinner, emphasizing whole foods and a variety of nutrients.

- Wind down with mobility exercises or relaxation techniques to promote quality sleep.

5. **Weekly Reflection:**
   - Designate a day each week for a comprehensive review of your workout journal.
   - Adjust your plan for the upcoming week based on your reflections, incorporating lessons learned and refining your approach.

In conclusion, monitoring progress is a dynamic process that involves meticulous documentation, strategic scheduling, and a flexible mindset. By maintaining a detailed workout journal, optimizing your daily schedule, and adjusting your plan as needed, you'll not only track progress but also ensure a sustainable and rewarding bodybuilding journey well into your 40s and beyond.

XI. Holistic Well-being and Longevity

A. Mental and Emotional Health

1. Mind-Body Connection:

- Explore the powerful connection between mental and physical well-being. Recognize the impact of stress on the body and implement strategies like mindfulness, meditation, or deep breathing exercises to promote mental resilience.

2. Goal Alignment:

- Reflect on the alignment of your fitness goals with your broader life objectives. Ensure that your bodybuilding journey contributes positively to your overall happiness, fulfillment, and life satisfaction.

B. Sleep Optimization

1. Importance of Quality Sleep:

- Delve into the critical role of sleep in muscle recovery, hormone regulation, and overall health. Understand the implications of inadequate sleep on performance and explore strategies to optimize sleep quality.

2. Sleep Hygiene Practices:

- Establish a sleep routine that includes practices such as maintaining a consistent sleep schedule, creating a conducive sleep environment, and minimizing electronic device usage before bedtime.

C. Stress Management

1. Stress and Its Impact:

- Examine the physiological effects of stress on the body and its potential to hinder progress in your bodybuilding journey. Implement stress management techniques to foster a healthier mind and body.

2. Adaptogenic Herbs and Supplements:

- Explore the potential benefits of adaptogenic herbs and supplements in mitigating the effects of stress. Consider incorporating adaptogens like ashwagandha or rhodiola into your routine under the guidance of a healthcare professional.

D. Hormonal Health

1. Age-Related Changes:

- Understand how hormonal changes associated with aging can influence muscle mass, metabolism, and overall vitality. Explore strategies to naturally support hormonal balance through lifestyle, nutrition, and exercise.

2. Hormonal Testing:

- Consider hormonal testing to assess baseline levels and identify any imbalances. Discuss the results with a healthcare provider to develop targeted interventions if necessary.

E. Community and Support

1. Importance of Community:

- Recognize the value of a supportive community in maintaining motivation and accountability. Whether through workout partners, online forums, or local fitness groups, fostering connections can enhance your overall fitness experience.

2. Seeking Professional Guidance:

- Consider engaging with fitness professionals, including personal trainers, nutritionists, and healthcare providers. Their expertise can provide personalized insights, address concerns, and optimize your bodybuilding plan for long-term success.

F. Adaptability and Resilience

1. Embracing Change:

- Acknowledge that fitness journeys evolve, and factors such as injuries, lifestyle shifts, or changing priorities may necessitate adjustments. Develop resilience and adaptability to navigate these changes while maintaining a commitment to your well-being.

2. Periodic Reassessment:

- Regularly reassess your fitness goals, preferences, and progress. Embrace the opportunity to recalibrate your workout plan, nutrition strategy, and overall approach to ensure continued growth and satisfaction.

G. Celebrating Milestones

1. Recognizing Achievements:

- Take time to acknowledge and celebrate your achievements, no matter how small. Reflecting on your progress boosts motivation and reinforces the positive habits contributing to your bodybuilding success.

2. Setting New Challenges:

- Continuously challenge yourself by setting new goals and aspirations. Whether it's conquering a new exercise, achieving a personal record, or mastering a new fitness skill, setting and pursuing challenges maintains excitement and momentum.

In this comprehensive chapter, we've explored the interconnected elements of holistic well-being and longevity in the context of bodybuilding for men above 40. By addressing mental and emotional health, optimizing sleep, managing stress, supporting hormonal balance, fostering community, embracing adaptability, and celebrating milestones, you'll cultivate a sustainable and fulfilling fitness journey that extends far beyond the gym.

BOOK SUMMARY

The journey begins with a purposeful introduction, emphasizing the importance of recognizing age-specific considerations and the necessity of consulting healthcare professionals before commencing the fitness endeavor. The guide systematically unfolds through ten chapters, each designed to provide a nuanced and practical approach to bodybuilding for mature individuals.

1. **Introduction:**
   - Emphasizes the need for a tailored approach, considering age-related changes and the significance of consulting healthcare professionals before starting the fitness journey.
2. **Warm-up and Mobility:**
   - Incorporates compelling stories to underscore the importance of a proper warm-up and dynamic stretching, ensuring joint health and

flexibility are prioritized in the workout routine.

3. **Resistance Training Phases:**

   - Divides the workout plan into foundational, strength development, and hypertrophy phases. It provides practical insights into choosing weights, incorporating intensity techniques, and optimizing recovery strategies.

4. **Cardiovascular Exercise:**

   - Stresses the importance of cardiovascular health, suggesting suitable activities, frequencies, and durations for effective results.

5. **Flexibility and Mobility:**

   - Introduces stretching, yoga, and myofascial release to enhance flexibility and joint health.

6. **Recovery and Rest:**

   - Highlights the significance of sleep, active recovery days, and incorporating rest weeks for overall recovery.

7. **Nutrition and Hydration:**

   - Emphasizes a balanced approach to nutrition, specifying the role of macronutrients and micronutrients. It also stresses the importance of hydration and offers guidance on suitable supplements.

8. **Protein Intake for Muscle Health:**

   - Utilizes a practical story to emphasize the individualized nature of protein needs, timing, and considerations for supplementation.

9. **Joint Health Supplements:**

   - Incorporates the stories of individuals like Steve, focusing on vitamins like Vitamin C and supplements like glucosamine and chondroitin to support joint health.

10. **Consultation with a Nutritionist:**

- Encourages seeking professional guidance for personalized nutrition plans, blood tests, and adjusting dosages for optimal benefits.

11. **Monitoring Progress:**

- Offers a comprehensive approach to tracking progress through workout journals, daily schedules, and a detailed plan. The chapter also underscores the importance of mental health, quality sleep, stress management, hormonal health, community support, and adaptability.

In conclusion, this guide is more than a workout plan; it's a lifestyle guide crafted for sustained success. By intertwining practical advice with compelling stories, the book navigates the intricate terrain of fitness for mature men, emphasizing not only physical strength but also mental resilience, emotional well-being, and a commitment to long-term health and longevity. Whether you are a seasoned fitness enthusiast or a novice, this guide serves as a holistic compass for achieving and sustaining strength beyond 40.